DIABETIC COOKBOOK

A Beginner's Guide to Tasty, Diabetes-Friendly Recipes

Transform Your Plate: Embrace Low Sugar, Low Carbs Recipes, Craft a Wholesome Meal Plan, and Cultivate Healthier Eating Habits.

ELLA WELLNESS

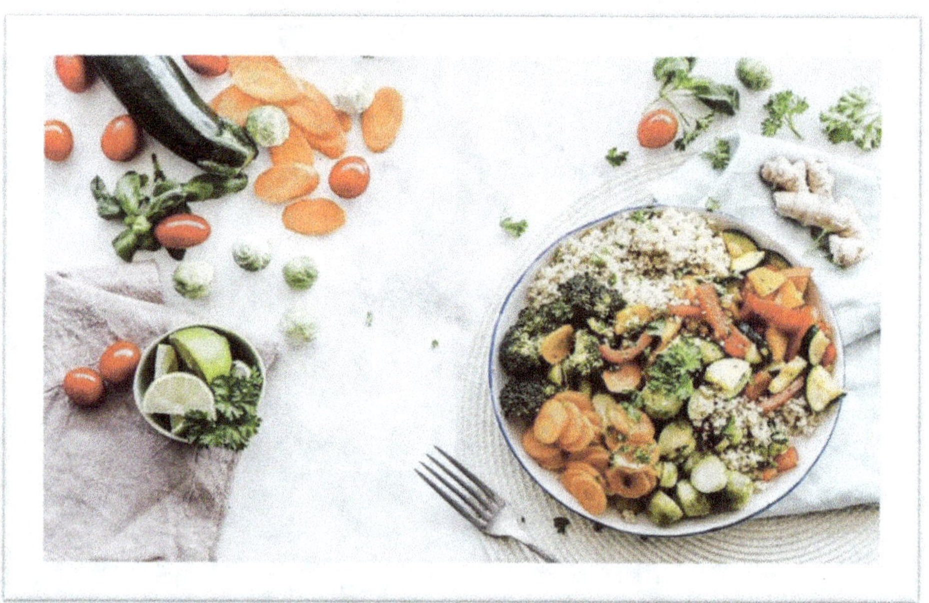

This book is intended to provide general information and guidance about diabetes-friendly recipes and healthier living. It is not intended as a substitute for professional medical advice or treatment. Always consult with your healthcare provider before making significant changes to your diet or lifestyle.

The recipes and information provided in this book have been carefully curated and are based on the author's research and knowledge up to the publication date. However, the author and publisher assume no responsibility for any errors, inaccuracies, omissions, or outcomes related to the use of this book.

Names, characters, places, and incidents mentioned in this book are purely the creation of the author's imagination and used fictitiously. Any resemblance to actual persons, living or dead, or real events is entirely coincidental.

DEDICATION

To all the brave souls who face each day with unwavering strength and courage, navigating the challenges of diabetes with resilience and hope.

May this book serve as a guiding light, illuminating the path to better health through delicious, diabetes-friendly recipes and valuable insights.

Your perseverance inspires us all, and it is an honour to contribute to your journey toward a sweeter balance in life.

With heartfelt admiration and support,

Table of Contents

Introduction..**5**

Chapter 1: Understanding Diabetes and Nutrition...**9**

Chapter 2: Transforming Your Breakfast...**17**

Chapter 3: Nourishing Lunches on the Go..**23**

Chapter 4: Satisfying Dinners for Every Palate..**32**

Chapter 5: Irresistible Diabetic-Friendly Desserts..**45**

Chapter 6: Smart Snacking for Diabetes Management..**66**

Chapter 7: Eating Out with Diabetes: Tips and Tricks for Smart Choices....................................**71**

Chapter 8: Mindful Eating: Building Healthy Habits...**74**

Chapter 9: Staying Active with Diabetes: Exercise and Fitness Tips.....................................**81**

Chapter 10: Diabetes Management and Blood Sugar Monitoring.......................................**84**

Chapter 11: Meal Planning and Grocery Shopping for Diabetes...**..**

Chapter 12: Managing Stress and Emotional

Eating……………………………………………………………………

Chapter 13: Incorporating Superfoods for Diabetes Health…………………………………………………….

Chapter 14: Cooking Techniques for Diabetes-Friendly Meals……………………………………………..

Chapter 15: Diabetic-Friendly Beverages and Hydration…………………………………………………………

Chapter 16: Special Occasion Menus and Holiday Treats

Conclusion

INTRODUCTION

Welcome to "Transform Your Plate: Embrace Low Sugar, Low Carbs Recipes, Craft a Wholesome Meal Plan, and Cultivate Healthier Eating Habits." This comprehensive diabetic cookbook is thoughtfully curated to empower individuals with diabetes, prediabetes, or those seeking a healthier lifestyle to take charge of their nutritional choices and optimize their well-being.

The prevalence of diabetes has been on the rise globally, becoming a significant health concern. According to the World Health Organization (WHO), approximately 422 million people were living with diabetes in 2021, and this number is projected to increase substantially in the coming years. Diabetes can have severe implications for an individual's health if not managed properly, leading to complications such as cardiovascular disease, kidney damage, nerve damage, and vision problems. However, the good news is that lifestyle modifications, particularly dietary changes, can play a vital role in diabetes management and overall health improvement.

Understanding the impact of nutrition on blood glucose levels is pivotal for those with diabetes. Carbohydrates, in particular, can cause significant fluctuations in blood sugar levels. Therefore, adopting a low sugar, low carb approach to cooking can be instrumental in managing diabetes and preventing sugar spikes. By reducing the consumption of sugary and high-carb foods, you can maintain more stable blood sugar levels, which contributes to better diabetes control and minimizes the risk of complications.

The primary focus of "Transform Your Plate" is to provide you with a diverse range of delicious recipes that are not only diabetes-friendly but also enjoyable for everyone, regardless of their dietary needs. Our culinary experts and nutritionists have carefully crafted these recipes to strike the perfect balance between taste and health, ensuring that you can still indulge in your favorite flavors without compromising your well-being.

Beyond the mouthwatering recipes, this cookbook equips you with valuable knowledge about diabetes and nutrition. Understanding the different types of diabetes, how carbohydrates impact blood glucose, and the significance of portion control can empower you to make informed decisions about your diet. By arming yourself with this knowledge, you can confidently navigate the grocery store aisles, read food labels critically, and select the most suitable ingredients for your meals.

Creating a diabetes-friendly pantry is a crucial step in adopting a healthier lifestyle. In "Transform Your Plate," we provide you with a comprehensive list of essential pantry items, including whole grains, healthy fats, and flavor-enhancing herbs and spices. Building a well-stocked pantry not only simplifies meal preparation but also ensures you always have the right ingredients on hand to whip up a nourishing and satisfying dish.

As you embark on this culinary journey, we also acknowledge that managing diabetes goes beyond just following recipes. Crafting a personalized diabetes meal plan tailored to your individual needs and lifestyle is paramount. With our guidance, you will learn how to create a balanced meal plan that incorporates a variety of nutrients and minimizes sugar and carb intake. This meal plan will not only aid in blood sugar control but also promote overall health and vitality.

Ultimately, "Transform Your Plate" is not solely focused on recipes; it's about cultivating healthier eating habits that last a lifetime. We believe that sustainable changes are rooted in mindfulness, portion awareness, and choosing nutrientdense, wholesome foods. Alongside the recipes, you will find tips and insights on mindful eating, portion control, and the importance of regular physical activity in managing diabetes and maintaining overall well-being.

EMBRACE THIS COOKBOOK AS A TOOL FOR TRANSFORMATIVE CHANGE, NOT JUST FOR YOUR PLATE BUT FOR YOUR ENTIRE LIFESTYLE. EACH MEAL YOU PREPARE HAS THE POWER TO NURTURE YOUR BODY, MIND, AND SPIRIT. TOGETHER, LET'S TAKE CHARGE OF OUR HEALTH, ONE DELICIOUS AND NUTRITIOUS RECIPE AT A TIME.

CHAPTER 1
UNDERSTANDING DIABETES AND NUTRITION

In this first chapter, "Understanding Diabetes and Nutrition," we embark on a journey to explore the core concepts that underpin diabetes and its profound connection to nutrition. Diabetes is a chronic condition that affects how the body processes glucose, a form of sugar that serves as a primary energy source. Properly managing diabetes requires a comprehensive understanding of how the foods we eat impact blood sugar levels. Whether you have recently been diagnosed with diabetes or have been living with the condition for some time, this chapter will provide you with valuable insights to support your journey towards healthier eating habits and better diabetes control.

Section 1: What is Diabetes?

Diabetes is a chronic medical condition that occurs when the body is unable to properly regulate blood glucose (sugar) levels. Glucose is a vital source of energy for the body, and its levels are tightly controlled by the hormone insulin, which is produced by the pancreas.

The Types of Diabetes:

Diabetes is a heterogeneous condition, and there are several types with distinct characteristics:

- Type 1 Diabetes: This autoimmune condition occurs when the body's immune system attacks and destroys the insulinproducing cells in the pancreas. As a result, individuals with Type 1 Diabetes must take insulin injections to manage their blood sugar levels effectively.

- Type 2 Diabetes: The most prevalent form of diabetes, Type 2 Diabetes, is primarily associated with lifestyle factors such as sedentary behavior, poor diet, and obesity. In Type 2 Diabetes, the body either resists the effects of insulin or doesn't produce enough insulin to maintain normal blood glucose levels.

Prediabetes: Prediabetes is a warning sign that blood sugar levels are higher than normal but not yet at the level of Type 2 Diabetes. It presents an opportunity for individuals to make lifestyle changes to prevent or delay the onset of diabetes.

Gestational Diabetes: Some women develop diabetes during pregnancy, known as gestational diabetes. Although it usually resolves after childbirth, it increases the risk of developing Type 2 Diabetes later in life.

Understanding Insulin:

Insulin is a hormone produced by the pancreas that facilitates the uptake of glucose from the bloodstream into cells, where it is used for energy.

In Type 1 Diabetes, the pancreas does not produce insulin, necessitating external insulin administration.

In Type 2 Diabetes, insulin resistance occurs, where the body's cells become less responsive to insulin, resulting in elevated blood sugar levels.

Proper insulin management is crucial for individuals with diabetes to regulate blood glucose effectively.

The Impact of Carbohydrates and Sugars on Blood Glucose

Carbohydrates and Blood Sugar Levels:

Carbohydrates are the primary macronutrient that influences blood sugar levels. They are broken down into glucose during digestion, leading to an increase in blood sugar levels.

Different types of carbohydrates have varying effects on blood glucose levels. Simple carbohydrates, such as those found in sugary beverages and candies, cause rapid spikes in blood sugar. On the other hand, complex carbohydrates, like those in whole grains and vegetables, are digested more slowly, leading to a gradual rise in blood glucose.

The Role of Sugars in Diabetes:

Sugars, particularly added sugars found in processed foods and sugary drinks, can contribute to blood sugar fluctuations, and negatively impact diabetes management.

It's essential for individuals with diabetes to be mindful of their sugar intake and choose natural sugar sources like fruits in moderation.

Section 3: Balancing Nutrients for Stable Blood Sugar Levels

The Importance of Balanced Meals:

Creating balanced meals that include a combination of carbohydrates, proteins, and healthy fats can help stabilize blood sugar levels and prevent drastic fluctuations.

Including protein and healthy fats in meals slows down the absorption of carbohydrates, leading to a more gradual rise in blood glucose.

The Power of Fiber:

Fiber is an essential component of a diabetes-friendly diet. It slows down the digestion and absorption of carbohydrates, leading to more stable blood sugar levels.

Foods rich in fiber, such as vegetables, fruits, whole grains, and legumes, are excellent choices for individuals with diabetes.

Portion Control and Meal Timing
Understanding Portion Sizes:

Controlling portion sizes is crucial for diabetes management, as it helps regulate blood sugar levels and manage weight.

Learning about appropriate portion sizes and practicing mindful eating can support better diabetes control.

Meal Timing and Frequency:

Spacing meals and snacks throughout the day can help prevent drastic blood sugar fluctuations and support steady energy levels.

Eating regular, balanced meals can also aid in weight management and improve insulin sensitivity.

Section 5: The Importance of Regular Physical Activity

Exercise and Diabetes Management:

Regular physical activity offers numerous benefits for individuals with diabetes, including improved insulin sensitivity, better blood sugar control, and weight management.

Exercise can also reduce the risk of cardiovascular complications associated with diabetes.

Finding enjoyable activities and incorporating them into daily life can increase adherence to an exercise routine.

Combining aerobic exercises, strength training, and flexibility exercises can provide a well-rounded approach to physical activity.

Understanding the intricate relationship between diabetes and nutrition is pivotal for effective diabetes management and overall well-being. By comprehending the impact of carbohydrates, sugars, and balanced meals on blood sugar levels, you can make informed dietary choices that support better diabetes control. Additionally, practicing portion control, meal timing, and incorporating regular physical activity can further enhance your efforts to manage diabetes successfully. As we progress through this cookbook, we will build on this knowledge and empower you to create flavorful, satisfying, and wholesome low sugar, low carb recipes that will transform your plate and nurture your health.

CHAPTER 2:

Building a Diabetes-Friendly Pantry

Introduction:

In Chapter 2, "Building a Diabetes-Friendly Pantry," we delve into the foundation of crafting wholesome and nourishing meals that support better diabetes management. A well-stocked pantry is essential for preparing diabetes-friendly dishes that are low in sugar, low in carbohydrates, and rich in nutrients. By carefully selecting the right ingredients, you can ensure that your culinary creations not only taste delicious but also contribute to stable blood sugar levels and overall health. Let's explore the key elements of building a pantry that empowers you to take charge of your diabetes through mindful and intentional food choices.

Section 1: The Essentials of a Diabetes-Friendly Pantry

1.1 Whole Grains and Grain Alternatives:

Whole grains are an excellent source of fiber, vitamins, and minerals. They have a lower glycemic index compared to refined grains, leading to more gradual increases in blood sugar levels.

Stock your pantry with whole grains such as brown rice, quinoa, barley, and whole wheat pasta, as well as grain alternatives like cauliflower rice and zucchini noodles.

1.2 Healthy Fats:

Healthy fats are an essential component of a diabetes-friendly diet. They help improve insulin sensitivity and promote heart health.

Include sources of healthy fats such as olive oil, avocado oil, nuts, seeds, and avocados in your pantry.

1.3 Flavor Enhancers:

Herbs and spices are a wonderful way to add depth and flavor to your dishes without relying on excessive salt or sugar.

Stock up on a variety of herbs and spices, such as cinnamon, turmeric, basil, rosemary, and garlic powder, to elevate the taste of your meals.

1.4 Low-Sugar Condiments:

Many store-bought condiments contain hidden sugars that can impact blood sugar levels. Opt for low-sugar or sugar-free alternatives for ketchup, BBQ sauce, and salad dressings.

Section 2: Identifying Hidden Sugars and High-Carb Ingredients

2.1 Reading Food Labels:
Understanding how to read food labels is vital for identifying hidden sugars and high-carb ingredients in packaged foods.
Look for words such as sucrose, high-fructose corn syrup, and maltodextrin, which indicate the presence of added sugars.

2.2 Making Informed Choices:

Learn to make informed choices by comparing different brands and products based on their nutritional content.

Look for products with lower sugar and carbohydrate content to support your diabetes management goals.

Section 3: Stocking up on Nutrient-Rich Ingredients

3.1 Powerhouse Vegetables:

Vegetables are packed with essential vitamins, minerals, and fiber. Aim to have a variety of fresh and frozen vegetables in your pantry, such as leafy greens, broccoli, bell peppers, and spinach.

3.2 Lean Proteins:

Including lean proteins in your meals helps stabilize blood sugar levels and supports muscle health.

Stock up on protein sources like skinless chicken breast, turkey, lean beef, fish, tofu, and legumes.

3.3 Low-Sugar Fruits:

While fruits contain natural sugars, some varieties are lower in sugar and make great additions to your pantry.

opt for berries, apples, citrus fruits, and melons, and enjoy them in moderation.

Section 4: Creating Diabetes-Friendly Staples

Homemade Sauces and Dressings:

Prepare your own sauces and dressings at home to control the sugar and carbohydrate content.

Experiment with simple recipes using ingredients from your pantry, such as homemade tomato sauce and vinaigrettes.

4.2 DIY Baking Mixes:

For occasional indulgences, create your own low-carb baking mixes using almond flour, coconut flour, and sugar substitutes.

Enjoy treats like sugar-free cookies and low-carb muffins without compromising your diabetes management.

A well-curated pantry is the foundation of a diabetes-friendly kitchen, offering you the tools to create delicious and wholesome meals that support your health goals. By stocking up on whole grains, healthy fats, flavor enhancers, and nutrient-rich ingredients, you can confidently prepare a diverse array of low sugar, low carb recipes that nurture your body and manage your diabetes effectively. Moreover, with an understanding of reading food labels and making informed choices, you can navigate the grocery store aisles with confidence, selecting products that align with your dietary needs. As we move forward in this cookbook, let's continue to leverage the power of a diabetes-friendly pantry and explore flavorful and nutritious recipes that will transform your plate and elevate your well-being.

CHAPTER 3

Introduction:

In Chapter 3, "Breakfasts to Start Your Day Right," we focus on the most important meal of the day and explore a variety of diabetes-friendly breakfast options that provide energy, satiety, and stable blood sugar levels. A balanced breakfast sets the tone for the rest of the day, and choosing low sugar, low carb recipes will support your diabetes management and promote overall well-being. From hearty and Savory dishes to satisfying sweet treats, this chapter offers a delightful assortment of breakfast ideas that cater to different tastes and dietary preferences.

Low Carb Smoothies and Protein-Packed Shakes

Berry-Banana Smoothie:

A refreshing and nutrient-rich smoothie made with berries, banana, unsweetened almond milk, and Greek yogurt.

Packed with antioxidants, vitamins, and protein, this smoothie is a delicious way to kick-start your day.

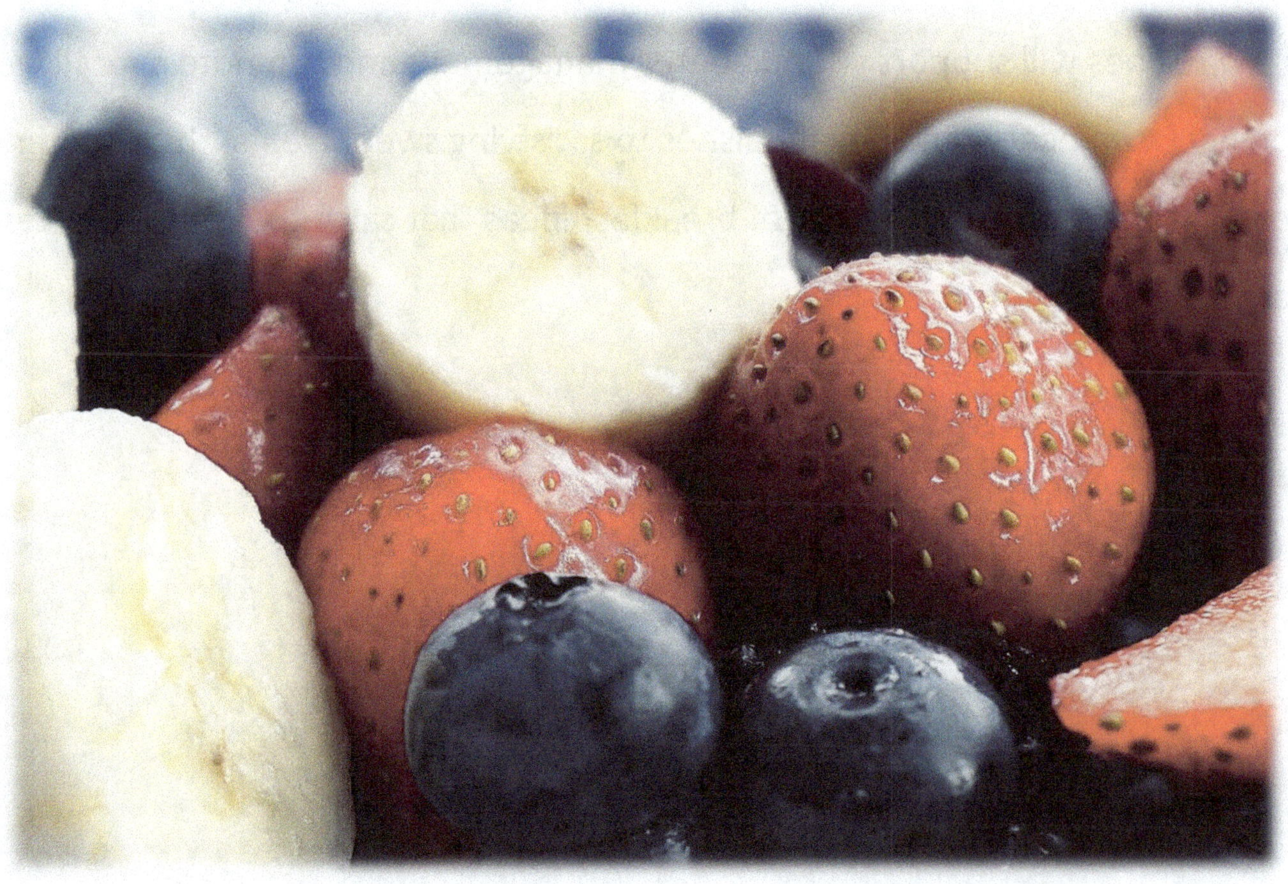

Chocolate Avocado Protein Shake:

A creamy and indulgent shake featuring avocado, unsweetened cocoa powder, protein powder, and almond milk.

Rich in healthy fats and protein, this shake keeps you full and satisfied until your next meal.

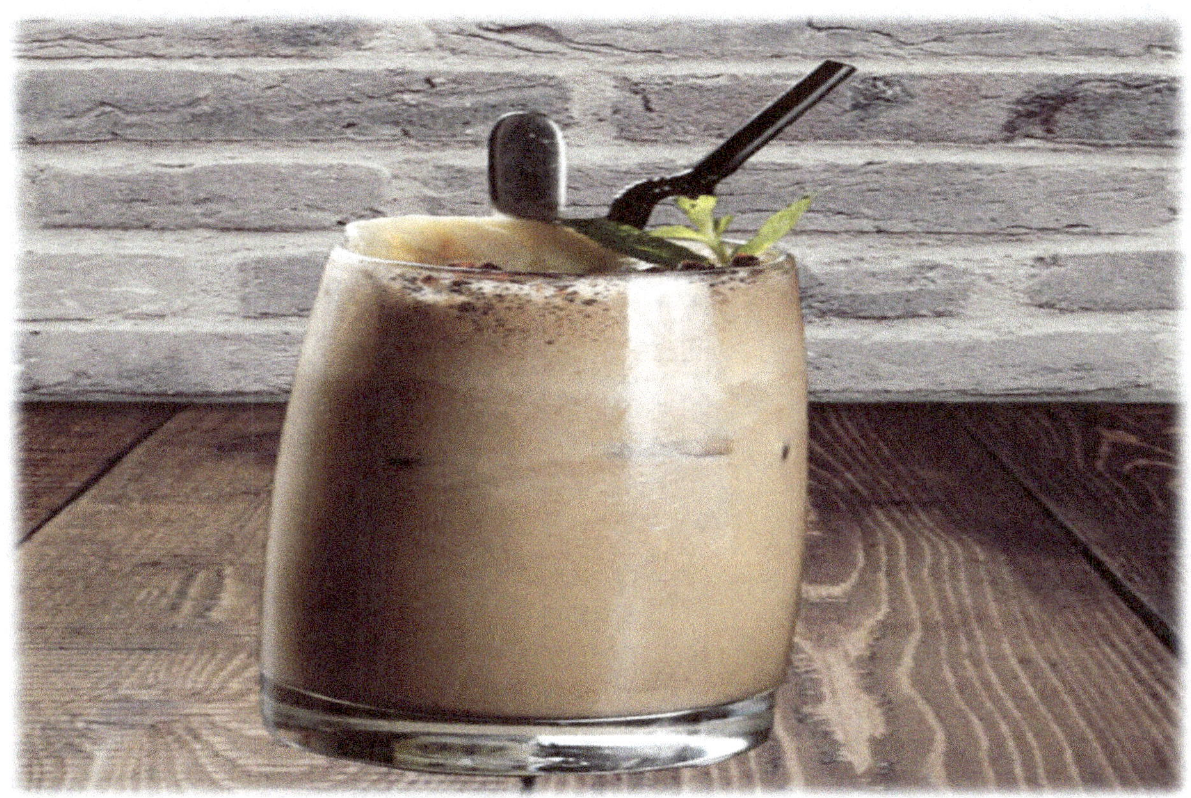

 Veggie Omelette:

A colourful omelette filled with a variety of sautéed vegetables such as bell peppers, spinach, and tomatoes.

High in fiber and low in carbs, this omelette is a nutrient-dense way to start your day.

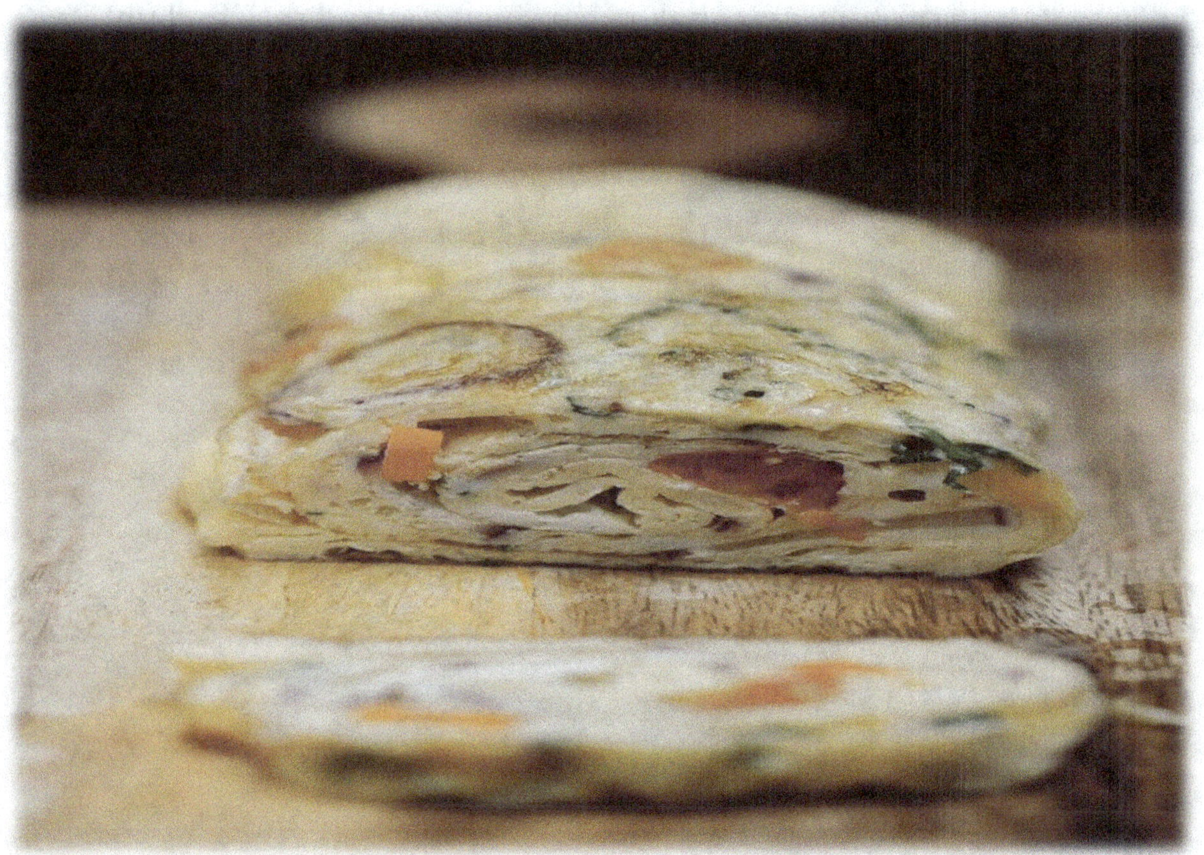

Spinach and Feta Scramble:

A savory scramble featuring spinach, feta cheese, and eggs, seasoned with herbs and spices.

This protein-packed dish provides essential nutrients and a burst of flavors.

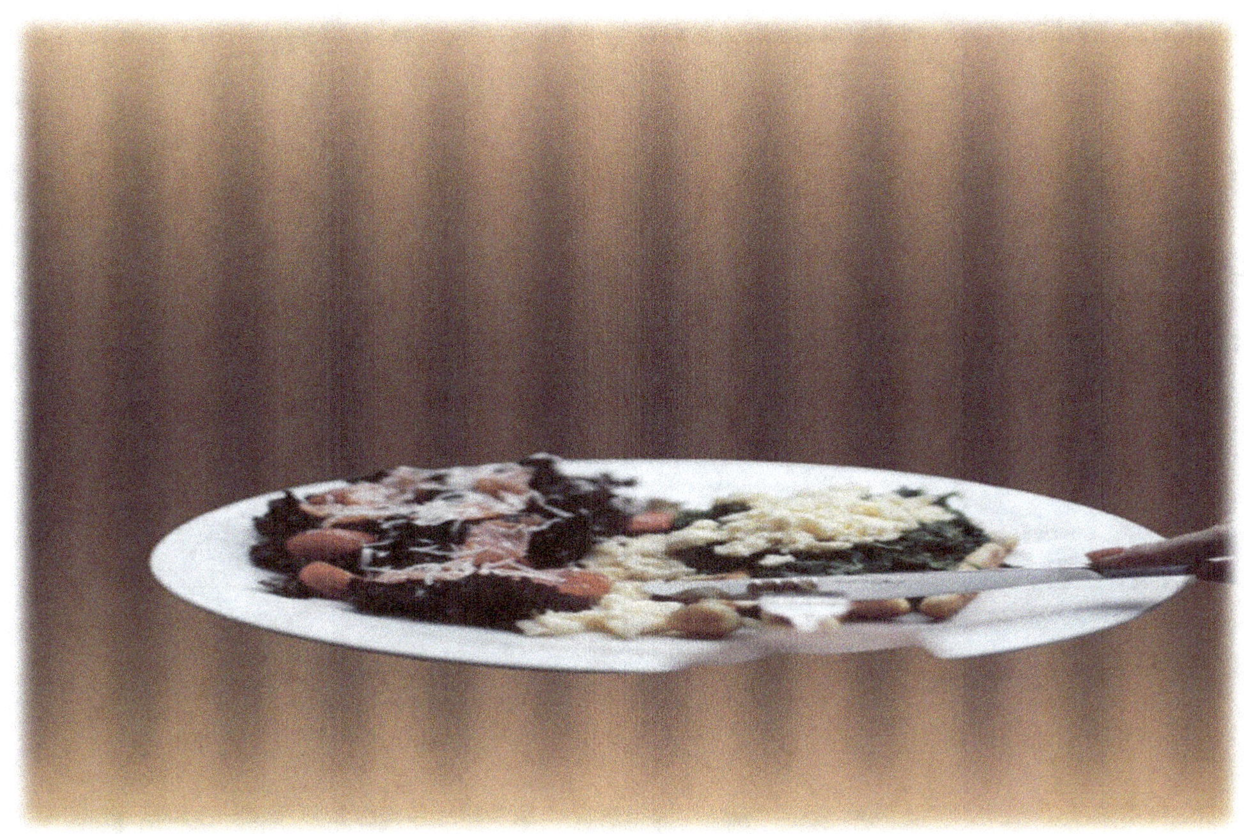

Wholesome Breakfast Bowls.

Start your day with a wholesome breakfast bowl packed with nourishment. Combine a base of creamy Greek yogurt or oatmeal with a medley of fresh fruits, nuts, and seeds for a delightful blend of flavors and textures. This nutritious bowl will provide you with a boost of energy and essential nutrients to kickstart your morning on a healthy note

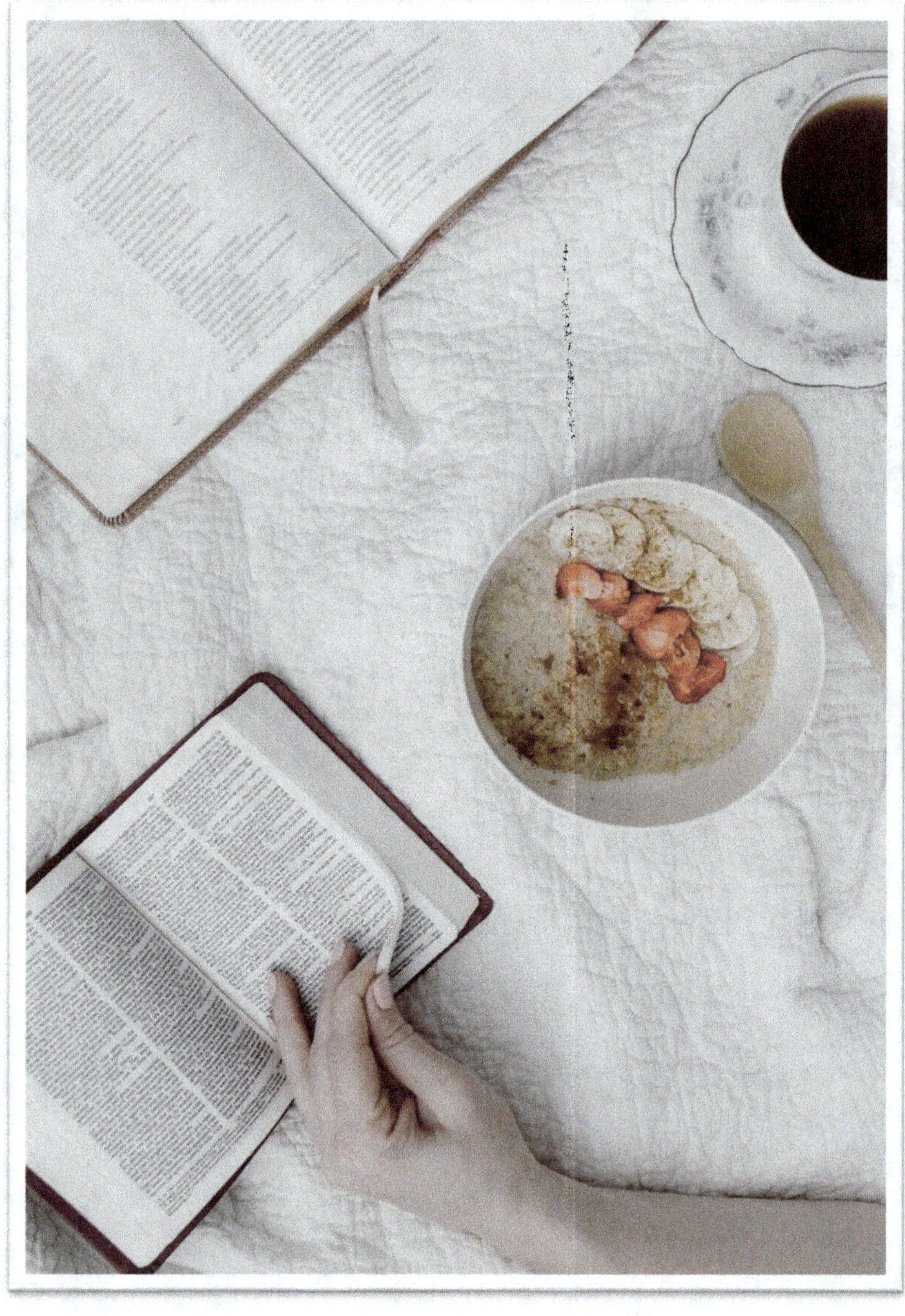

Quinoa Breakfast Bowl:

A nourishing bowl of cooked quinoa topped with fresh fruits, nuts, and a drizzle of honey (optional).

Quinoa offers a complete protein source and is low on the glycaemic index, making it an excellent choice for stable blood sugar levels.

3.2 Chia Seed Pudding:

A creamy and satisfying chia seed pudding made with chia seeds, unsweetened almond milk, and a touch of vanilla extract.

Chia seeds are rich in fiber, omega-3 fatty acids, and protein, making this pudding a nutritious morning

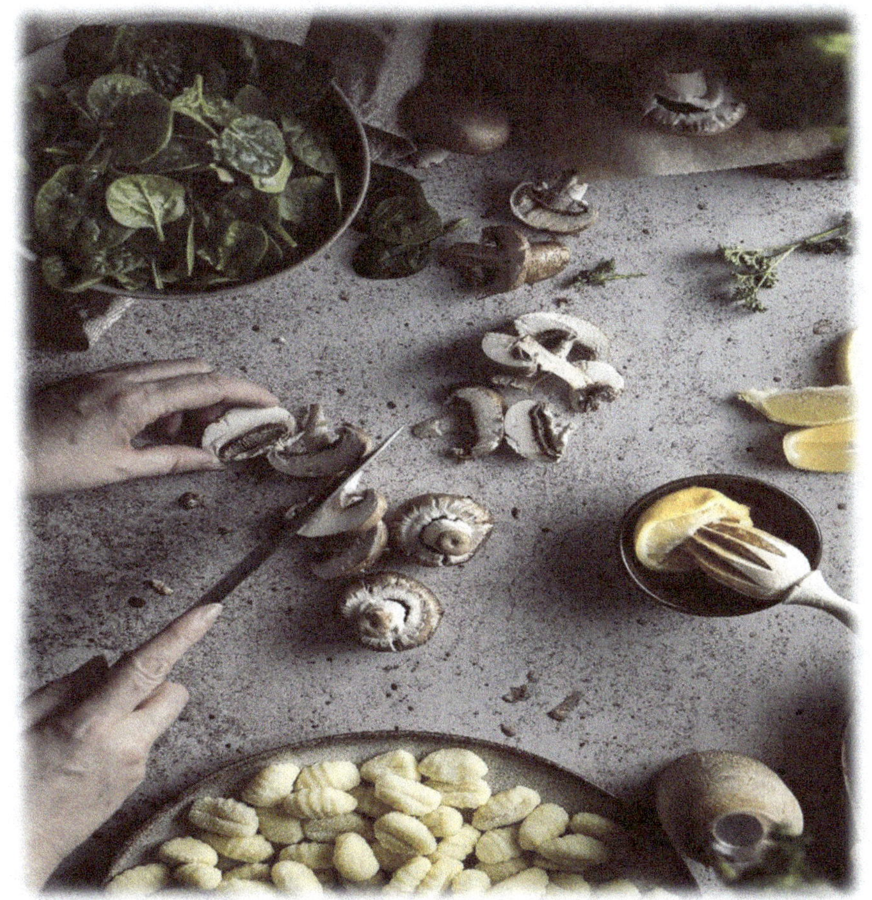

treat.

Hearty Vegetable Frittatas

4.1 Mushroom and Spinach Frittata:

A hearty frittata filled with mushrooms, spinach, onions, and a sprinkle of low-fat cheese.

Frittatas are an excellent way to incorporate vegetables and protein into your breakfast.

Mediterranean Frittata:

A Mediterranean-inspired frittata featuring cherry tomatoes, olives, feta cheese, and fresh herbs.

This flavorful frittata is a delightful departure from traditional breakfast fare.

Section 5: Breakfasts on the Go

Low-Carb Breakfast Muffins:

Savory muffins made with almond flour, eggs, and a variety of vegetables and herbs.

These portable muffins are perfect for busy mornings or as a quick snack.

Peanut Butter and Banana Wrap:

A simple and delicious wrap made with whole-grain tortillas, natural peanut butter, and sliced bananas.

This easy-to-assemble wrap is a great option for those on the move.

Conclusion:

Starting your day with a diabetes-friendly breakfast is the key to setting yourself up for success. In this chapter, we have explored a diverse range of breakfast options that cater to various tastes and dietary needs. From nutrient-rich smoothies and protein-packed shakes to satisfying egg dishes, wholesome breakfast bowls, and hearty vegetable frittatas, these recipes provide a myriad of flavors and textures that will keep you excited about breakfast every day.

By choosing low sugar, low carb breakfasts, you can maintain stable blood sugar levels, feel more energized, and support your diabetes management journey. Additionally, these breakfast options are packed with essential nutrients, fiber, and protein, making them not only delicious but also nourishing for your body.

As you experiment with these recipes, feel free to customize them to suit your taste preferences and dietary requirements. With "Breakfasts to Start Your Day Right," you can embrace a healthy and satisfying morning routine that will set the stage for a day filled with vitality and well-being. Let's continue our culinary exploration in the following chapters, crafting more diabetes-friendly recipes that will transform your plate and enhance your quality of life.

CHAPTER 4:

Nourishing Lunches on the Go Introduction:

In Chapter 4, "Nourishing Lunches on the Go," we focus on creating
diabetesfriendly lunch options that are not only delicious and satisfying but also
convenient for those with busy schedules. Whether you're heading to work,
school, or simply looking for quick and nutritious lunch ideas, this chapter offers
a diverse array of recipes that will keep you energized throughout the day.
These lunch options are designed to be low in sugar, low in carbohydrates, and
rich in essential nutrients, making them ideal for maintaining stable blood sugar
levels and supporting your overall health and well-being

➢ Grilled Chicken and Avocado Salad:

A refreshing salad featuring grilled chicken, avocado, mixed greens, cherry tomatoes, and a tangy vinaigrette dressing.

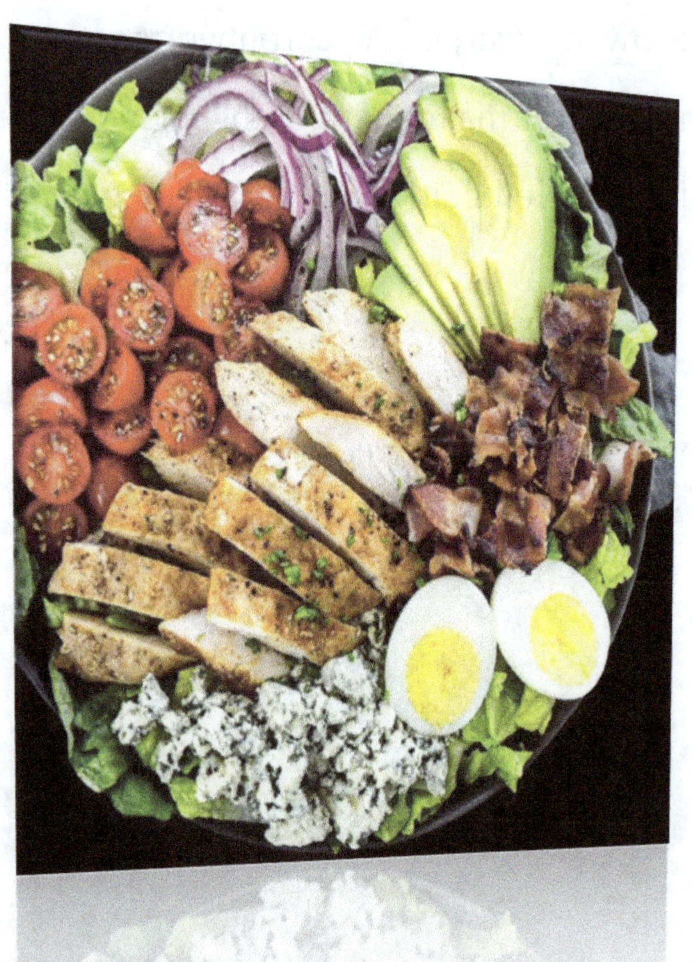

High in protein, healthy fats, and fiber, this salad keeps you satiated and nourished.

• Quinoa and Roasted Vegetable Salad:

A hearty salad made with cooked quinoa, roasted vegetables, feta cheese, and a light lemon herb dressing.

Quinoa provides a complete protein source, while the roasted veggies add a burst of flavor and nutrition.

Section 2: Wholesome Wraps and Sandwiches

• Turkey and Hummus Wrap:

A satisfying wrap filled with lean turkey slices, hummus, cucumber, lettuce, and a sprinkle of feta cheese.

This wrap is a delicious combination of protein, healthy fats, and fresh vegetables.

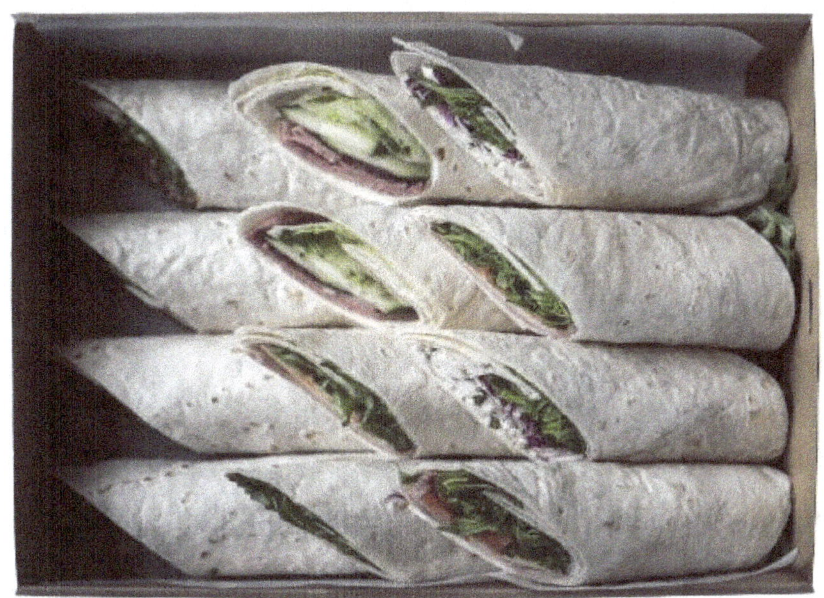

- Veggie and Avocado Sandwich:

A delightful sandwich with whole-grain bread, sliced avocado, cucumber, bell peppers, and a smear of low-fat cream cheese.

Packed with vitamins, minerals, and healthy fats, this sandwich offers a nourishing lunch option.

Section 3: Hearty and Satisfying Soups

- Lentil and Vegetable Soup:

A comforting and filling soup made with lentils, a variety of vegetables, and aromatic herbs and spices.

Lentils provide a good source of plant-based protein and fiber, making this soup a diabetes-friendly choice.

- Chicken and Vegetable Soup

A classic chicken soup featuring tender chicken, carrots, celery, and onions in a flavorful broth.

This soup is a comforting option that provides essential nutrients and supports hydration.

1 pound (450g) boneless, skinless chicken breasts or thighs, diced

1 tablespoon olive oil

1 medium onion, finely chopped

2 garlic cloves, minced

2 medium carrots, sliced

2 celery stalks, sliced

1 medium zucchini, diced

1 cup fresh or frozen green beans, cut into 1-inch pieces

1 can (14 ounces) diced tomatoes

6 cups chicken broth or stock

1 teaspoon dried thyme

1 teaspoon dried oregano

Salt and pepper to taste

Fresh parsley for garnish (optional)

Instructions:

- Heat the Oil

- In a large pot or Dutch oven, heat the olive oil over medium heat.

- Sauté Onion and Garlic:

- Add the chopped onion and minced garlic to the pot. Sauté for 2-3 minutes until the onion becomes translucent and fragrant.

- Add Chicken:

- Add the diced chicken to the pot and cook until it's lightly browned on all sides. This should take about 5 minutes.

- Add Vegetables:

- Now, add the sliced carrots, celery, diced zucchini, and green beans to the pot. Stir everything together and cook for another 5 minutes to soften the vegetables slightly.

- Pour in Tomatoes and Broth

- Pour in the can of diced tomatoes with their juices and the chicken broth or stock. Stir in the dried thyme and oregano.

- Season and Simmer

- Season the soup with salt and pepper to taste. Bring the mixture to a boil, then reduce the heat to low, cover the pot with a lid, and let it simmer for about 15-20 minutes or until the vegetables are tender and the chicken is fully cooked.

- Adjust Seasoning
- Taste the soup and adjust the seasoning as needed with more salt and pepper, if desired.

- Serve

Ladle the hot Chicken and Vegetable Soup into serving bowls. Garnish with fresh parsley, if desired, for added flavor and presentation.

Enjoy!

Serve the soup hot and enjoy a delicious and comforting meal.

Note: Feel free to customize the soup by adding other favorite vegetables, such as peas, corn, or spinach, to suit your taste preferences. You can also

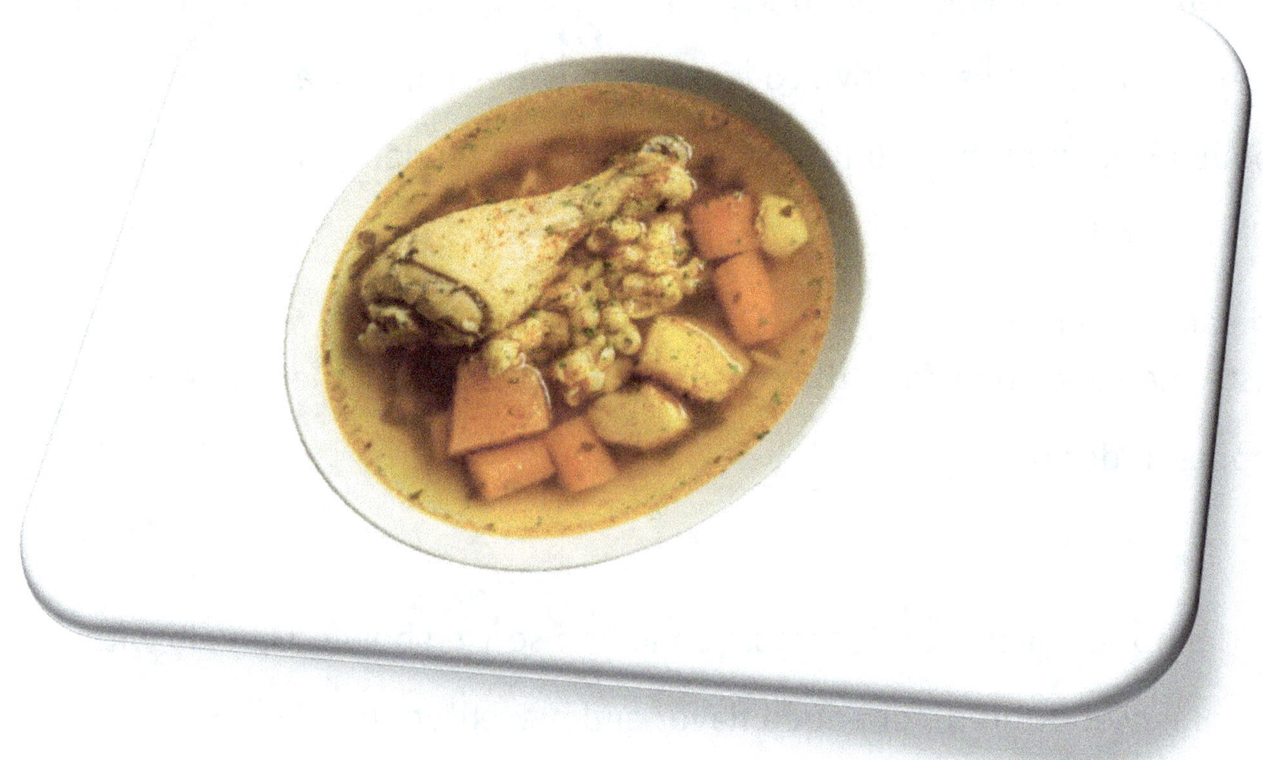

experiment with different herbs and spices to create unique variations of this wholesome soup.

Protein-Packed Bowls

4.1 Shrimp and Avocado Bowl:

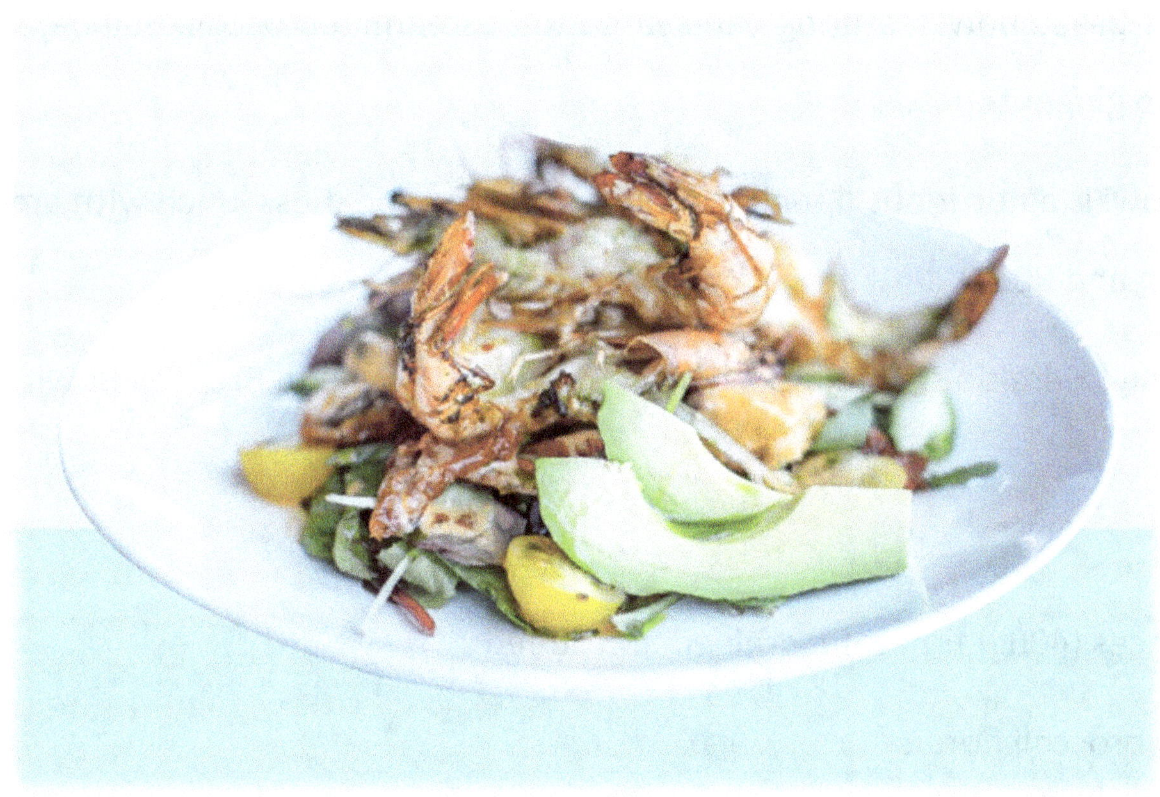

A protein-packed bowl with grilled shrimp, avocado slices, brown rice, black beans, and a drizzle of lime dressing.

This bowl offers a delightful combination of flavors and textures with a balance of protein and healthy fats.

▪ Tofu and Broccoli Bowl:

A plant-based bowl featuring pan-seared tofu, steamed broccoli, quinoa, and a sesame ginger sauce.

This bowl is a nutritious option for those seeking a meatless lunch with ample protein and fiber.

Certainly! Here's a simple procedure to prepare a Tofu and Broccoli Bowl:

Ingredients:

14 ounces (400g) firm tofu, drained and cubed

2 cups broccoli florets

1 tablespoon soy sauce or tamari (for a gluten-free option)

1 tablespoon sesame oil

2 cloves garlic, minced

1 tablespoon grated fresh ginger

2 tablespoons vegetable oil (for frying tofu)

Cooked rice or quinoa (for serving)

Sesame seeds and sliced green onions for garnish (optional)

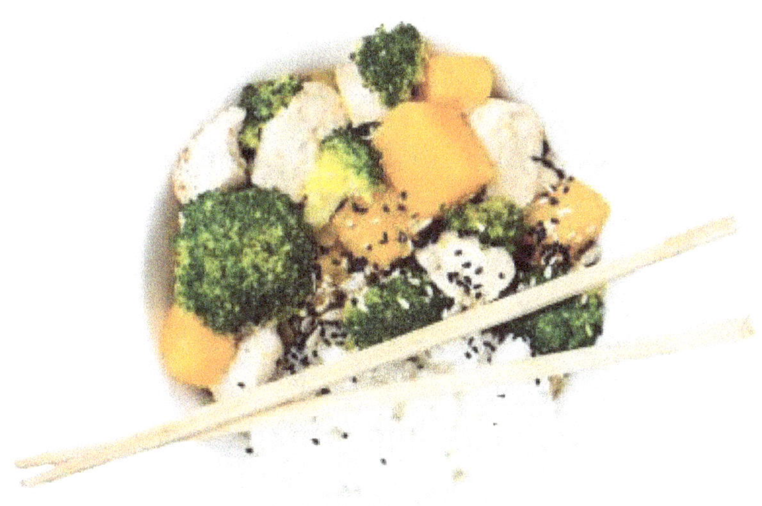

Instructions:

- Marinate the Tofu:

In a bowl, mix the cubed tofu with soy sauce (or tamari) and sesame oil.
Allow the tofu to marinate for at least 10-15 minutes to absorb the flavors.

- Blanch the Broccoli:
- Bring a pot of water to a boil and add the broccoli florets. Blanch the broccoli for 1-2 minutes until it turns bright green and slightly tender. Remove the broccoli from the boiling water and immediately place it in a bowl of ice water to stop the cooking process. Drain and set aside.

- Fry the Tofu:

In a large skillet or pan, heat the vegetable oil over medium heat. Add the marinated tofu cubes to the hot oil and fry until they become golden and crispy on all sides. This should take about 5-7 minutes. Remove the fried tofu from the pan and set it aside.

- Sauté Garlic and Ginger:

In the same skillet, add minced garlic and grated ginger. Sauté for about 1 minute until the aroma is released and the garlic turns slightly golden.

- Add Broccoli and Tofu:

Return the blanched broccoli to the skillet, along with the fried tofu. Toss everything together to combine and heat the ingredients evenly.

- Serve:

Serve the Tofu and Broccoli over cooked rice or quinoa in bowls. You can drizzle any remaining marinade over the bowl for extra flavor. Garnish with sesame seeds and sliced green onions, if desired, for added texture and presentation.

Enjoy!

Enjoy your delicious and nutritious Tofu and Broccoli Bowl, packed with protein, fiber, and a delightful blend of Asian-inspired flavors. This dish makes for a satisfying and wholesome meal that's quick and easy to prepare.

Portable Snack Boxes

- Bento Box with a Variety of Snacks:

A versatile bento box filled with an assortment of snacks like cheese cubes, mixed nuts, cherry tomatoes, and sliced fruits.

Bento boxes are perfect for those who prefer grazing throughout the day or want to enjoy a diverse range of flavors.

- Greek Yogurt Parfait:

A delightful and nutritious parfait made with Greek yogurt, berries, and a sprinkle of granola.

This parfait is a quick and easy option for a satisfying and balanced lunch.

Conclusion:

In "Nourishing Lunches on the Go," we have explored a selection of diabetesfriendly lunch ideas that cater to different tastes and lifestyles. From fresh and flavorful salads to wholesome wraps, hearty soups, protein-packed bowls, and portable snack boxes, these recipes offer a diverse array of options to suit your preferences.

Preparing low sugar, low carb lunches ensure stable blood sugar levels and provides a steady source of energy throughout the day. Additionally, these lunch options are rich in essential nutrients, fiber, and protein, making them nourish for your body and supporting your diabetes management journey.

By incorporating these recipes into your lunch routine, you can enjoy convenient and delicious meals that contribute to your overall well-being. With "Nourishing Lunches on the Go," you can take charge of your midday nourishment and elevate your lunchtime experience. As we continue our culinary exploration in the following chapters, we will further uncover delightful recipes that will transform your plate and inspire healthier eating habits.

Introduction:

In Chapter 5, "Satisfying Dinners for Every Palate," we invite you to discover a delightful collection of diabetes-friendly dinner options that cater to diverse tastes and dietary preferences. These recipes are designed to be both flavorful and wholesome, ensuring that individuals with diabetes can enjoy delicious dinners while maintaining stable blood sugar levels and supporting overall health. From classic comfort foods to international delights, this chapter offers a culinary journey that will transform your dinner table into a haven of culinary pleasure and nourishment.

Classic Comfort Foods

Baked Lemon Herb Salmon

Ingredients:

2 salmon fillets

2 tablespoons fresh lemon juice

1 tablespoon olive oil

1 teaspoon dried thyme

1 teaspoon dried rosemary

Salt and pepper to taste

Instructions:

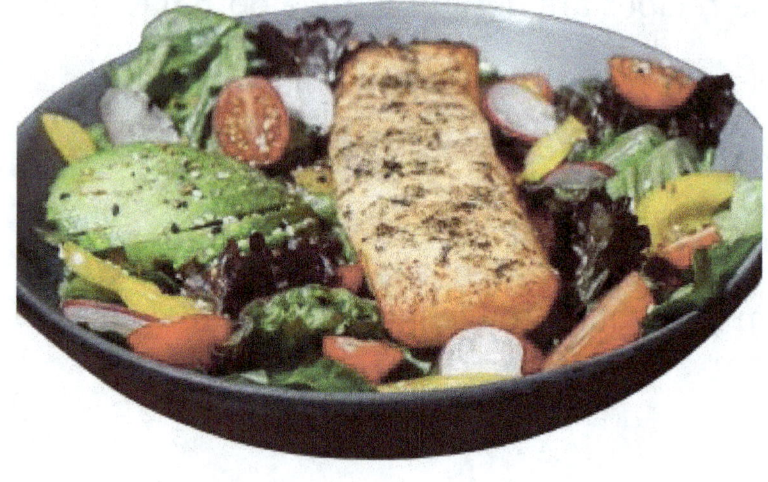

Preheat the oven to 375°F (190°C) and line a baking sheet with parchment paper.

In a small bowl, whisk together the lemon juice, olive oil, dried thyme, dried rosemary, salt, and pepper.

Place the salmon fillets on the prepared baking sheet, and brush the lemon herb mixture over each fillet.

Bake the salmon in the preheated oven for 12-15 minutes or until the salmon is cooked through and

flakes easily with a fork.

Serve the baked lemon herb salmon with a side of steamed vegetables or a fresh salad for a delicious and hearthealthy dinner.

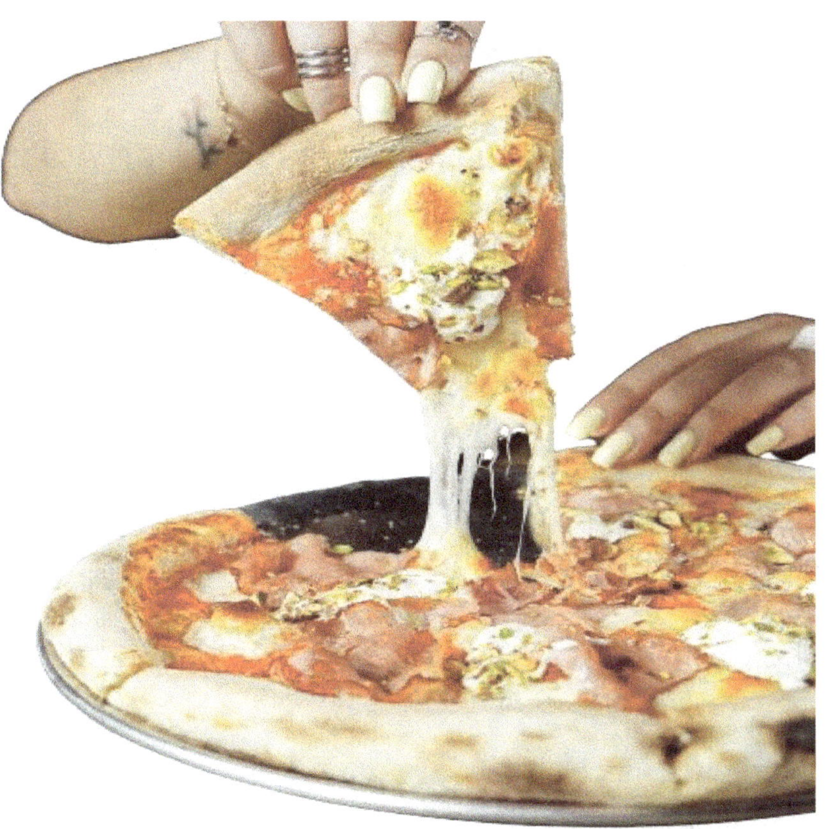

Cauliflower Crust Pizza

Ingredients:

1 medium cauliflower head, grated

1 large egg, beaten

1/2 cup shredded mozzarella cheese (part-skim)

1 teaspoon dried oregano

1/2 teaspoon garlic powder

1/4 cup pizza sauce (sugar-free or low-sugar) Assorted vegetable toppings (bell peppers, onions, mushrooms, etc.) 1/4 cup shredded low-fat mozzarella cheese (for topping)

Instructions:

Preheat the oven to 425°F (220°C) and line a baking sheet with parchment paper.

In a microwave-safe bowl, microwave the grated cauliflower for 4-5 minutes until softened. Let it cool slightly.

Using a clean kitchen towel or cheesecloth, squeeze out as much moisture as possible from the cooked cauliflower.

In a mixing bowl, combine the cauliflower, beaten egg, shredded mozzarella cheese, dried oregano, and garlic powder. Mix well to form a dough-like consistency.

Place the cauliflower dough on the prepared baking sheet and shape it into a circular pizza crust, about 1/4 inch thick.

Bake the crust in the preheated oven for 20-25 minutes or until golden brown and crisp around the edges.

Remove the crust from the oven and spread pizza sauce over it. Add your preferred vegetable toppings and sprinkle low-fat mozzarella cheese over the top.

Return the pizza to the oven and bake for an additional 8-10 minutes or until the cheese is melted and bubbly.

Let the cauliflower crust pizza cool slightly before slicing and serving. Enjoy this guilt-free and delicious pizza for a satisfying dinner option.

International Delights

Thai Basil Chicken Stir-Fry

Ingredients:

2 boneless, skinless chicken breasts, thinly sliced

2 tablespoons vegetable oil

3 garlic cloves, minced

1 red bell pepper, sliced

1 yellow bell pepper, sliced

1 cup sliced green beans

2 tablespoons soy sauce (low-sodium)

1 tablespoon oyster sauce (or fish sauce for a saltier option)

1 tablespoon hoisin sauce

1 tablespoon brown sugar or a sugar substitute

1 cup fresh basil leaves

Cooked brown rice (for serving)

Instructions:

In a wok or large skillet, heat the vegetable oil over medium-high heat.

Add the minced garlic and sauté for about 30 seconds until fragrant.

Add the sliced chicken breasts and stir-fry until cooked through and lightly browned.

Add the sliced bell peppers and green beans to the wok and continue stirfrying for 2-3 minutes until the vegetables are tender-crisp.

In a small bowl, whisk together the soy sauce, oyster sauce, hoisin sauce, and brown sugar.

Pour the sauce over the chicken and vegetables in the wok. Stir-fry for an additional 1-2 minutes until everything is coated in the sauce.

Remove the wok from the heat and stir in the fresh basil leaves.

Serve the Thai basil chicken stir-fry over cooked brown rice for a delightful and aromatic dinner inspired by the flavors of Thailand.

Greek Spinach and Feta Stuffed Peppers

Ingredients:

4 large bell peppers (red, yellow, or orange)

1 tablespoon olive oil

1 medium onion, finely chopped

2 garlic cloves, minced

2 cups fresh spinach leaves, chopped

1 cup cooked quinoa

1/2 cup crumbled feta cheese

1 teaspoon dried oregano

Salt and pepper to taste

Instructions:

Preheat the oven to 375°F (190°C) and line a baking dish with parchment paper.

Cut the tops off the bell peppers and remove the seeds and membranes. Set aside.

In a large skillet, heat the olive oil over medium heat. Add the chopped onion and minced garlic, and sauté until the onion becomes translucent.

Add the chopped spinach to the skillet and cook until wilted.

Stir in the cooked quinoa, crumbled feta cheese, dried oregano, salt, and pepper. Mix everything until well combined.

Stuff each bell pepper with the quinoa mixture, pressing down gently to pack it in.

Place the stuffed bell peppers in the prepared baking dish and bake in the preheated oven for 25-30 minutes or until the peppers are tender and lightly browned on the edges.

Remove the stuffed peppers from the oven and let them cool slightly before serving. Enjoy these Greek-inspired stuffed peppers as a flavorful and nutritious dinner option.

Vegetarian and Plant-Based Dinners

Eggplant Parmesan Ingredients:

1 large eggplant, sliced into rounds

2 cups marinara sauce (sugar-free or low-sugar)

1 cup shredded mozzarella cheese (part-skim)

1/2 cup grated Parmesan cheese

1 cup whole wheat breadcrumbs

2 tablespoons chopped fresh basil

2 tablespoons chopped fresh parsley

Salt and pepper to taste

Olive oil cooking spray

Instructions:

Preheat the oven to 375°F (190°C) and line a baking sheet with parchment paper.

Arrange the eggplant slices on the baking sheet in a single layer. Lightly spray the eggplant slices with olive oil cooking spray and season with salt and pepper.

Bake the eggplant slices in the preheated oven for 20 minutes or until tender and slightly golden.

In a small bowl, mix the whole wheat breadcrumbs, chopped fresh basil, chopped fresh parsley, and grated Parmesan cheese to make the breadcrumb mixture.

In a greased baking dish, layer half of the baked eggplant slices. Top the eggplant with half of the marinara sauce, half of the shredded mozzarella cheese, and half of the breadcrumb mixture.

Repeat the layers with the remaining eggplant, marinara sauce, mozzarella cheese, and breadcrumb mixture.

Bake the eggplant Parmesan in the preheated oven for 20-25 minutes or until the cheese is melted and bubbly, and the breadcrumbs are golden brown.

Let the eggplant Parmesan cool for a few minutes before serving. Enjoy this vegetarian twist on a classic Italian favorite as a comforting and satisfying dinner option.

Lentil and Vegetable Curry

Ingredients:

1 cup dried green lentils, rinsed

1 tablespoon vegetable oil

1 medium onion, chopped

2 garlic cloves, minced

1 tablespoon grated ginger

1 tablespoon curry powder

1 teaspoon ground cumin

1 teaspoon ground turmeric

1/2 teaspoon ground coriander

1/4 teaspoon cayenne pepper (adjust to your spice preference)

1 can (14 oz) diced tomatoes (low-sodium if possible)

1 can (13.5 oz) coconut milk (light or full-fat)

2 cups mixed vegetables (carrots, bell peppers, zucchini, etc.)

Salt and pepper to taste

Fresh cilantro for garnish

Cooked brown rice or quinoa (for serving)

Instructions:

In a medium saucepan, bring 2 cups of water to a boil. Add the rinsed lentils and a pinch of salt. Reduce heat to low, cover, and simmer for 15-20 minutes or until the lentils are tender. Drain any excess water and set aside.

In a large skillet or pot, heat the vegetable oil over medium heat. Add the chopped onion and sauté until translucent.

Stir in the minced garlic and grated ginger, and cook for another minute until fragrant.

Add the curry powder, ground cumin, ground turmeric, ground coriander, and cayenne pepper to the skillet. Stir to coat the onions and spices evenly.

Pour in the diced tomatoes (with their juices) and coconut milk. Bring the mixture to a simmer, and let it cook for about 5 minutes.

Add the mixed vegetables to the curry sauce and continue to simmer for an additional 5 minutes or until the vegetables are tender.

Stir in the cooked lentils and season the curry with salt and pepper to taste.

Serve the lentil and vegetable curry over cooked brown rice or quinoa. Garnish with fresh cilantro for added flavor and color. Enjoy this hearty and aromatic plant-based curry for a nutritious and satisfying dinner.

Comforting One-Pot Meals

Hearty Chicken and Vegetable Soup

Ingredients:

2 boneless, skinless chicken breasts, cut into bite-sized pieces

1 tablespoon vegetable oil

1 medium onion, chopped

2 garlic cloves, minced

2 carrots, peeled and chopped

2 celery stalks, chopped

1 cup chopped green beans

1 can (14 oz) diced tomatoes (low-sodium if possible)

4 cups low-sodium chicken broth

2 cups water

1 teaspoon dried thyme

1 bay leaf

Salt and pepper to taste

Fresh parsley for garnish

Instructions:

In a large pot or Dutch oven, heat the vegetable oil over medium heat. Add the chopped onion and sauté until translucent.

Stir in the minced garlic and cook for another minute until fragrant.

Add the bite-sized chicken pieces to the pot and cook until lightly browned on all sides.

Add the chopped carrots, celery, and green beans to the pot. Stir everything together and cook for a few minutes until the vegetables start to soften.

Pour in the diced tomatoes (with their juices), chicken broth, and water. Stir in the dried thyme and bay leaf.

Bring the soup to a boil, then reduce the heat to low, cover the pot, and let it simmer for about 20 minutes or until the chicken is cooked through and the vegetables are tender.

Season the soup with salt and pepper to taste.

Ladle the hearty chicken and vegetable soup into bowls, and garnish with fresh parsley for added freshness and flavor. Enjoy this comforting and nourishing one-pot meal for a satisfying dinner.

Quinoa and Black Bean Chili

Ingredients:

1 cup quinoa, rinsed.

1 tablespoon vegetable oil

1 medium onion, chopped.

2 garlic cloves, minced

1 red bell pepper, chopped.

1 yellow bell pepper, chopped

1 can (14 oz) diced tomatoes (low-sodium if possible)

2 cans (15 oz each) black beans, drained and rinsed

1 cup low-sodium vegetable broth or water

2 tablespoons chili powder

1 teaspoon ground cumin

1/2 teaspoon smoked paprika

Salt and pepper to taste

Fresh cilantro and sliced green onions for garnish

Instructions:

In a medium saucepan, bring 2 cups of water to a boil. Add the rinsed quinoa and a pinch of salt. Reduce heat to low, cover, and simmer for 15-20 minutes or until the quinoa is cooked and the water is absorbed. Fluff with a fork and set aside.

In a large pot or Dutch oven, heat the vegetable oil over medium heat. Add the chopped onion and sauté until translucent.

Stir in the minced garlic and cook for another minute until fragrant.

Add the chopped red bell pepper and yellow bell pepper to the pot. Cook for a few minutes until the peppers start to soften.

Pour in the diced tomatoes (with their juices), black beans, and vegetable broth or water. Stir in the chili powder, ground cumin, smoked paprika, salt, and pepper.

Bring the chili to a simmer and let it cook for about 15-20 minutes to allow the flavors to meld together.

Stir in the cooked quinoa to the chili and let it simmer for an additional 5 minutes.

Ladle the quinoa and black bean chili into bowls, and garnish with fresh cilantro and sliced green onions for added freshness and flavour. Enjoy this hearty and protein-packed one-pot meal as a satisfying dinner option.

- Portobello Mushroom Steaks:

Juicy and savoury Portobello mushroom caps marinated in balsamic vinegar and grilled to perfection.

These mushroom steaks are a delicious option for those seeking a meatless dinner with a satisfying texture.

Ingredients:

4 large Portobello mushroom caps

3 tablespoons balsamic vinegar

2 tablespoons olive oil

2 garlic cloves, minced

Salt and pepper to taste

Instructions:

Preheat the grill or grill pan over medium-high heat.

In a small bowl, whisk together the balsamic vinegar, olive oil, minced garlic, salt, and pepper.

Brush the balsamic marinade over the Portobello mushroom caps, coating them evenly on both sides.

Place the mushroom caps on the grill or grill pan and cook for about 5-6 minutes on each side or until the mushrooms are tender and lightly charred.

Remove the Portobello mushroom steaks from the grill and let them rest for a few minutes before serving.

Serve the grilled Portobello mushroom steaks with a side of mixed greens or a fresh salad for a delicious and meatless dinner option.

- Zucchini Noodles with Pesto Sauce:

A light and refreshing dinner featuring zucchini noodles tossed in a vibrant homemade pesto sauce.

This dish offers a low-carb alternative to traditional pasta with a burst of herbaceous flavours.

Ingredients:
4 medium zucchinis, spiralized or thinly sliced into noodles

1 cup fresh basil leaves

1/4 cup pine nuts

1/4 cup grated Parmesan cheese

2 garlic cloves

1/3 cup extra-virgin olive oil

Salt and pepper to taste

Cherry tomatoes and extra grated Parmesan cheese for garnish

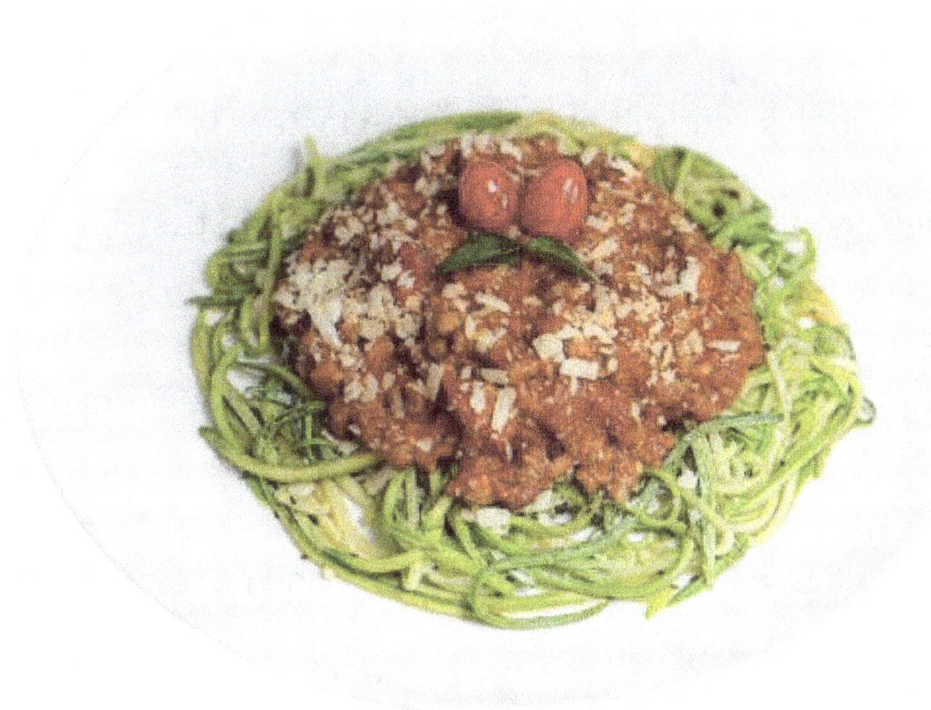

Instructions:

In a blender or food processor, combine the fresh basil leaves, pine nuts, grated Parmesan cheese, garlic cloves, and extra-virgin olive oil. Blend until a smooth and creamy pesto sauce forms.

In a large skillet, heat a tablespoon of olive oil over medium heat. Add the zucchini noodles and sauté for 2-3 minutes until they are just tender.

Stir in the prepared pesto sauce, coating the zucchini noodles evenly with the sauce.

Season the zucchini noodles with salt and pepper to taste.

Remove the zucchini noodles with pesto from the skillet and transfer them to a serving platter.

Garnish the dish with halved cherry tomatoes and extra grated Parmesan cheese for added color and flavor.

Serve the zucchini noodles with pesto sauce as a light and refreshing dinner option that is low in carbs and high in flavor.

Conclusion:

In "Satisfying Dinners for Every Palate," we have explored an enticing variety of diabetes-friendly dinner options that will elevate your evening meals to new heights of pleasure. Whether you crave classic comfort foods, desire to explore international delights, enjoy vegetarian and plant-based meals, or prefer comforting one-pot dishes, these recipes cater to diverse tastes and dietary needs.

Preparing low sugar, low carb dinners ensures stable blood sugar levels and supports your diabetes management journey. Additionally, these dinner options are rich in essential nutrients, proteins, and healthy fats, making them satisfying and nourishing for your body.

With these delightful recipes, dinner will become a time of culinary enjoyment and a chance to connect with loved ones over nourishing and wholesome meals. As we continue our culinary journey in the following chapters, we will explore more delightful recipes that will transform your plate and inspire a lifetime of healthier eating habits.

In Chapter 6, "Irresistible Diabetic-Friendly Desserts," we venture into the realm of delectable sweet treats that cater to individuals with diabetes without compromising on taste or satisfaction. Desserts are a delightful part of any meal, and with careful ingredient selection, we can create mouthwatering treats that are low in sugar and carbohydrates while still being indulgent. From creamy and luscious to fruity and refreshing, this chapter offers a delightful array of diabetic-friendly desserts that will satisfy your sweet cravings without causing drastic spikes in blood sugar levels.

Decadent and Creamy Delights

- Avocado Chocolate Mousse:

A velvety and rich chocolate mousse made with ripe avocados, unsweetened cocoa powder, and a touch of sweetener.

Avocados provide healthy fats and creamy texture, creating a guilt-free and luxurious dessert.

- Greek Yogurt Panna Cotta:

A smooth and creamy panna cotta made with Greek yogurt, gelatin, and a hint of vanilla extract.

This elegant dessert is a delightful way to end a meal on a light and refreshing note.

Fruity and Nutty Creations

- Berry Chia Seed Pudding:

A delightful chia seed pudding layered with a medley of fresh berries and a drizzle of honey (optional).

Chia seeds offer a wealth of fiber and nutrients, making this dessert both satisfying and nutritious.

- Baked Apples with Cinnamon and Walnuts:

Warm and tender baked apples topped with a sprinkle of cinnamon and toasted walnuts.

This cozy dessert is reminiscent of apple pie without the excessive sugar and carbs.

Frozen Delights

- Mixed Berry Frozen Yogurt:

A refreshing frozen yogurt featuring a blend of mixed berries, Greek yogurt, and a touch of stevia or sugar substitute.

Enjoy the sweetness of berries without the added sugars, perfect for a cool and guilt-free dessert.

- Chocolate-Dipped Banana Bites:

Frozen banana slices dipped in dark chocolate and sprinkled with chopped nuts or coconut flakes.

These delightful bites offer a satisfying combination of creamy banana and indulgent chocolate.

Wholesome Baked Treats

- Almond Flour Blueberry Muffins:

Moist and flavourful blueberry muffins made with almond flour, eggs, and fresh blueberries.

These muffins are a delightful low-carb alternative to traditional bakery muffins.

    ❑ Flourless Lemon Almond Cake:

A light and zesty cake made with almond meal and fresh lemon zest, sweetened with a sugar substitute.

This flourless cake is perfect for those who prefer gluten-free desserts. Section 5: Guilt-Free Pies and Crumbles

    ❑ Mini Mixed Berry Pies with Oat Crust:

Individual-sized mixed berry pies with a wholesome oat crust and a touch of natural sweetener.

These mini pies are bursting with fruity flavors and are perfect for portion control.

    ❑ Apple Cinnamon Crumble:

Baked apples topped with a cinnamon-infused crumble made with almond flour and a sugar substitute.

This comforting dessert will fill your home with the aroma of baked apples and warm spices.

Conclusion:

In "Irresistible Diabetic-Friendly Desserts," we have explored an array of sweet indulgences that cater to individuals with diabetes, offering a delightful way to enjoy desserts without compromising on health. These desserts are crafted with ingredients that are low in sugar and carbohydrates, ensuring stable blood sugar levels while satisfying your sweet tooth.

From creamy avocado chocolate mousse to fruity berry chia seed pudding and refreshing frozen yogurt, these desserts offer a diverse range of flavors and textures to suit every palate. Moreover, the use of wholesome ingredients like almond flour, Greek yogurt, fresh fruits, and natural sweeteners provides added nutritional value to these treats.

With these irresistible diabetic-friendly desserts, you can enjoy the pleasure of sweet indulgence while supporting your diabetes management journey. As we continue our culinary exploration in the following chapters, we will uncover more delightful recipes that will transform your plate and inspire you to embrace a lifetime of healthier and satisfying eating habits.

CHAPTER 7:
Smart Snacking for Diabetes Management

Introduction:

In Chapter 7, "Smart Snacking for Diabetes Management," we delve into the world of nutritious and diabetes-friendly snacks that help regulate blood sugar levels, curb hunger, and provide sustained energy throughout the day. Snacking plays a crucial role in maintaining stable blood sugar levels and preventing overeating during main meals. By choosing smart and balanced snacks that are low in sugar and carbs but rich in essential nutrients, individuals with diabetes can support their health goals and successfully manage their condition. This chapter presents a variety of delicious and satisfying snack ideas to keep you nourished and energized between meals.

Fresh and Flavourful Fruit Snacks

 Apple Slices with Peanut Butter:

Crisp apple slices paired with natural peanut butter for a delightful combination of sweet and savoury flavours.

Apples provide fibre, vitamins, and minerals, while peanut butter adds protein and healthy fats.

☐ Berries and Greek Yogurt Parfait:

A refreshing parfait made with mixed berries, Greek yogurt, and a sprinkle of granola or nuts.

Berries are low in sugar and high in antioxidants, making them an excellent choice for a guilt-free snack.

Wholesome Veggie Delights

☐ Carrot Sticks with Hummus:

Crunchy carrot sticks served with creamy hummus for a satisfying and nutrient-packed snack.

Carrots offer a dose of beta-carotene and fibre, while hummus provides protein and healthy fats.

☐ Cucumber and Cottage Cheese Bites:

Sliced cucumber rounds topped with cottage cheese and a sprinkle of herbs or spices.

This refreshing snack is low in carbs and a good source of hydration. Section 3: Protein-Packed Snacks

 Hard-Boiled Eggs

Protein-rich hard-boiled eggs seasoned with a pinch of salt and pepper for a quick and convenient snack.

Eggs provide a complete source of protein and essential nutrients.

3.2 Turkey and Cheese Roll-Ups:

Slices of lean turkey rolled up with low-fat cheese for a portable and satisfying snack.

These roll-ups are an excellent source of protein and can be customized with different types of cheese.

- Mixed Nuts

A handful of mixed nuts, such as almonds, walnuts, and pistachios, for a crunchy and heart-healthy snack.

Nuts are rich in healthy fats, protein, and fiber, promoting a sense of fullness and supporting heart health.

- Roasted Chickpeas:

Crunchy roasted chickpeas seasoned with spices like paprika or cumin for a flavorful and nutritious snack.

Chickpeas offer a combination of protein and fiber, making them a satisfying option.

Creative and Quick Snacks

- Rice Cake with Avocado and Tomato:

A rice cake topped with creamy avocado slices and fresh tomato for a simple and tasty snack.

Avocado provides healthy fats, while the rice cake offers a light and crispy base.

- Mini Caprese Skewers:

Mini skewers with cherry tomatoes, mozzarella balls, and fresh basil leaves for a delightful and colourful snack.

This snack is a low-carb twist on the classic Caprese salad.

In "Smart Snacking for Diabetes Management," we have explored an array of nutritious and delicious snack ideas that cater to individuals with diabetes. Smart snacking is a vital component of diabetes management, providing sustained energy, curbing hunger, and supporting stable blood sugar levels. These snacks are thoughtfully crafted to be low in sugar and carbohydrates while offering a balance of protein, healthy fats, and essential nutrients.

By incorporating these smart snack options into your daily routine, you can nourish your body, maintain your energy levels, and effectively manage your diabetes. Additionally, these snacks are convenient and easy to prepare, making them perfect for on-the-go or at-home enjoyment.

With these diabetes-friendly snacks, you can indulge in tasty treats that align with your health goals. As we conclude this chapter and continue our culinary exploration, let's further uncover delightful recipes that will transform your plate and inspire you to embrace a lifetime of healthier snacking habits.

Introduction:

In Chapter 8, "Eating Out with Diabetes: Tips and Tricks for Smart Choices," we navigate the world of dining out while effectively managing diabetes. Eating out at restaurants, cafes, and other food establishments can present challenges for individuals with diabetes due to the potential hidden sugars, high-carb options, and large portion sizes. However, with the right knowledge and strategies, you can make smart choices that align with your dietary needs and support your diabetes management goals. This chapter provides valuable tips and tricks to help you enjoy dining out without compromising your health.

Preparing for Dining Out

Reviewing Menus in Advance:

Before heading to a restaurant, review the menu online to identify diabetesfriendly options.

Look for dishes that are low in sugar, moderate in carbs, and include lean proteins and vegetables.

Planning Snacks Ahead of Time:

If you anticipate a long wait before the meal arrives, have a small, healthy snack before leaving home to prevent overeating or succumbing to unhealthy choices.

Making Informed Menu Choices

Opting for Protein-Based Dishes:

Choose dishes centered around lean proteins like grilled chicken, fish, or tofu.

Protein helps stabilize blood sugar levels and keeps you feeling full and satisfied.

Focusing on Vegetables:

Request extra vegetables or side salads to fill your plate with fiber-rich and nutrient-packed options.

Vegetables can help balance the meal and reduce the impact of carbohydrates.

Managing Carbohydrates

Choosing Whole Grains:

If possible, opt for whole grain options like brown rice, quinoa, or whole wheat pasta.

Whole grains have a lower glycemic index and provide more nutrients compared to refined grains.

Controlling Portions:

Be mindful of portion sizes, especially for high-carb dishes like pasta and bread.

Consider sharing a meal or asking for a to-go box to save half for another meal.

Navigating Hidden Sugars

Requesting Sauces and Dressings on the Side:

Request sauces and dressings on the side to control the amount you use.

Many sauces and dressings contain hidden sugars that can impact blood sugar levels.

Avoiding Sweetened Beverages:

Opt for water, unsweetened tea, or beverages without added sugars.

Sweetened beverages can lead to rapid spikes in blood sugar levels.

Managing Dessert Temptations

Sharing Desserts:

If you crave dessert, consider sharing with others at the table to enjoy a taste without overindulging.

Sharing desserts can also create a social and enjoyable dining experience.

Choosing Lower-Sugar Options:

Look for desserts that are naturally lower in sugar, such as fresh fruit or a cheese plate.

Alternatively, opt for diabetic-friendly desserts, like those mentioned in Chapter 6.

In "Eating Out with Diabetes: Tips and Tricks for Smart Choices," we have explored valuable strategies to help you navigate dining out with diabetes successfully. By planning ahead, making informed menu choices, managing carbohydrates, and being mindful of hidden sugars, you can enjoy meals at restaurants while prioritizing your health and well-being.

Eating out doesn't have to be a challenge when you have the right knowledge and tools to make smart choices. With the tips and tricks provided in this chapter, you can confidently enjoy dining out while effectively managing your diabetes. Remember that moderation and balance are key, and making healthier choices most of the time will contribute to your long-term diabetes management goals.

As we conclude this chapter and continue our journey towards a healthier lifestyle, let's explore further insights and delicious recipes that will transform your plate and empower you to embrace a fulfilling and diabetesfriendly dining experience.

CHAPTER 9:
Mindful Eating: Building Healthy Habits

In Chapter 9, we explore the transformative practice of mindful eating and its profound impact on fostering a positive and sustainable relationship with food. Mindful eating is all about being fully present during meals, understanding hunger and fullness cues, and consciously making choices that nourish the body. By embracing mindful eating, individuals can prevent overeating, make healthier food decisions, and effectively support their diabetes management journey, all while cultivating a profound appreciation for the pleasures of food.

The Basics of Mindful Eating:

☐ Being Present at Meals:

Before diving into a meal, it's crucial to take a moment to connect with the senses and be fully present with the food. Engaging all senses, including sight, smell, taste, and texture, allows one to fully experience the joy of eating and appreciate the culinary delights before them.

☐ Recognizing Hunger and Fullness:

Mindful eating encourages actively listening to the body's cues for hunger and fullness. By tuning into these internal signals, individuals can ascertain when to start and stop eating, ultimately fostering a more intuitive and balanced approach to nourishment. Eliminating distractions such as television or smartphones while eating is instrumental in staying in touch with these essential cues.

 Making Conscious Food Choices:

Nourishing the body with nutrient-dense foods is vital for overall well-being. Choosing a balanced variety of foods such as fruits, vegetables, whole grains, lean proteins, and healthy fats supports optimal health and energy levels. By making these conscious food choices, individuals can sustain a wholesome diet that promotes their overall health and diabetes management.

 Savoring Each Bite:

Mindful eaters take the time to savor each mouthful. By chewing food thoroughly and mindfully appreciating the flavors and textures, individuals enhance their connection with the eating experience. Eating slowly aids in improving digestion and increasing overall satisfaction with the meal, leading to a greater sense of contentment and satiety.

☐ Recognizing Emotional Triggers:

An essential aspect of mindful eating involves acknowledging emotional triggers that may lead to overeating or unhealthy indulgence. By cultivating self-awareness, individuals can identify patterns of emotional eating and develop strategies to manage these triggers effectively.

☐ Practicing Mindful Coping Techniques:

Mindful coping techniques play a crucial role in managing emotional eating. Engaging in stress-reducing activities like meditation, deep breathing exercises, or engaging hobbies can help individuals redirect their emotional responses away from food.

Conclusion:

Chapter 9 illuminates the transformative power of mindful eating, guiding individuals towards building healthier eating habits. By being fully present, recognizing hunger and fullness cues, making conscious food choices, and managing emotional eating triggers, one can embrace a balanced and nourishing approach to food that supports overall well-being and diabetes management. In the journey of mindful eating, individuals will discover a profound appreciation for the pleasures of food and a newfound sense of empowerment in their relationship with nourishment.

CHAPTER 10

Introduction:

Chapter 10, "Staying Active with Diabetes: Exercise and Fitness Tips," focuses on the importance of regular physical activity for individuals with diabetes. Exercise plays a vital role in managing blood sugar levels, improving insulin sensitivity, and promoting cardiovascular health. In this chapter, we explore various exercise options, provide fitness tips, and emphasize the significance of incorporating physical activity into daily routines to support diabetes management and overall well-being.

Understanding the Benefits of Exercise for Diabetes

 Blood Sugar Management:

Regular physical activity helps lower blood sugar levels and improve insulin sensitivity.

Engaging in exercise can reduce the need for diabetes medications and insulin doses.

 Cardiovascular Health:

Exercise supports heart health by reducing the risk of cardiovascular complications associated with diabetes.

It helps lower blood pressure and cholesterol levels, promoting overall cardiovascular well-being.

Exercise Options for Diabetes

- Aerobic Exercise:

Activities such as brisk walking, jogging, cycling, swimming, and dancing improve cardiovascular fitness and aid in blood sugar regulation.

Aim for at least 150 minutes of moderate aerobic activity or 75 minutes of vigorous activity per week.

- Strength Training:

Resistance exercises, such as weightlifting and bodyweight exercises, build muscle mass and enhance insulin sensitivity.

Include strength training activities at least two days per week.

Section 3: Exercise Safety and Monitoring

- Blood Sugar Monitoring:

Check blood sugar levels before, during, and after exercise, especially when trying a new activity or adjusting diabetes medications.

Monitoring blood sugar helps prevent hypoglycemia (low blood sugar) or hyperglycemia (high blood sugar) during physical activity.

- Staying Hydrated:

Drink plenty of water before, during, and after exercise to maintain proper hydration levels.

Proper hydration supports optimal exercise performance and helps regulate blood sugar levels.

Tips for Staying Motivated

- Setting Realistic Goals:

Set achievable and measurable exercise goals to stay motivated and track progress.

Celebrate small milestones to stay encouraged on your fitness journey.

- Finding Enjoyable Activities:

Engage in physical activities you enjoy, whether it's dancing, hiking, playing sports, or taking group fitness classes.

Enjoyable activities are more likely to become long-term habits.

Conclusion:

Chapter 10 highlights the significance of staying active with diabetes and incorporating regular exercise into daily routines. By understanding the benefits of exercise, exploring various exercise options, and prioritizing safety and monitoring, individuals can effectively manage blood sugar levels and promote cardiovascular health. Staying motivated through realistic goalsetting and enjoyable activities ensures that exercise becomes a sustainable and fulfilling part of a diabetes management plan. With a combination of regular physical activity, mindful eating, and smart choices when dining out, individuals with diabetes can lead active, healthy lives and empower themselves to thrive in their diabetes management journey.

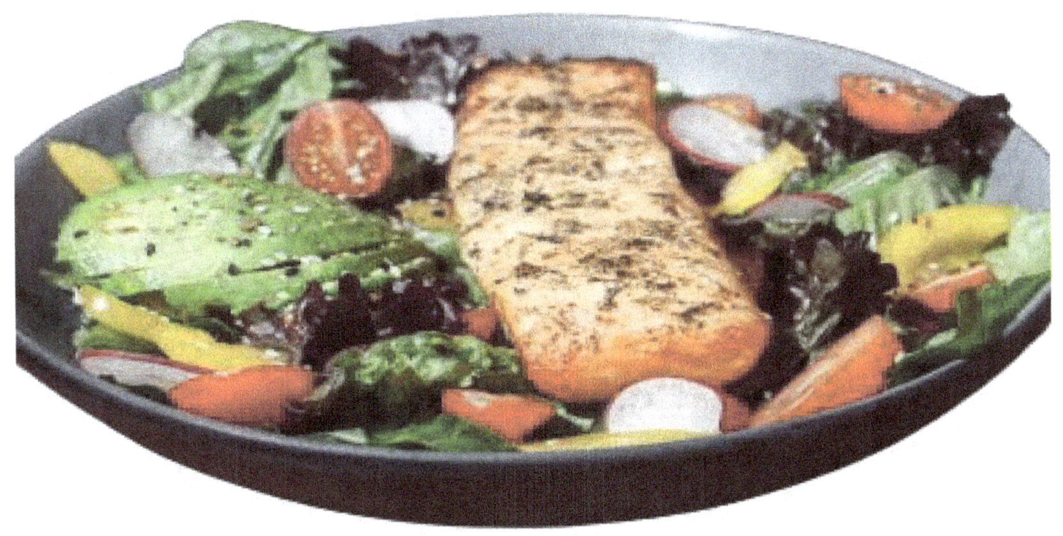

CHAPTER 11

Meal Planning and Grocery Shopping for Diabetes

In Chapter 11, we explore the vital aspects of meal planning and grocery shopping for individuals with diabetes. These practices are essential for managing blood sugar levels and promoting overall health. By creating wellbalanced meals and making informed choices at the grocery store, you can ensure that your diet supports your diabetes management goals. Let's dive into practical tips and strategies that will enable you to craft diabetesfriendly meal plans and build a well-stocked, nutritious pantry.

Meal Planning Basics:

Understanding the Importance of Meal Planning

Benefits of Structured Meal Planning for Blood Sugar Control and Health

Creating Balanced Meals:

The Plate Method: Building Balanced and Healthy Meals

Counting Carbs for Diabetes Management

The Glycemic Index and Glycemic Load

Building a Diabetes-Friendly Grocery List:

Stocking Up on Nutrient-Rich Foods Avoiding High-Sugar and High-Carb Foods

Smart Grocery Shopping Tips:

Preparing for Grocery Shopping Success

Exploring the Perimeter of the Grocery Store

Choosing Whole Foods and Minimally Processed Options

Reading Food Labels Wisely

Meal Prepping for Success:

The Benefits of Meal Prepping for Diabetes Management

Planning and Batch Cooking Proper

Storage and Portion Control

Conclusion:

In Chapter 11, we've explored the significance of meal planning and grocery shopping for individuals with diabetes. By understanding the fundamentals of balanced meals, carb counting, and glycemic impact, you can create a diabetes-friendly grocery list that supports your health and wellness goals. Armed with smart grocery shopping tips and meal prepping strategies, you can make informed choices and ensure that your kitchen is stocked with nourishing and wholesome ingredients. As you adopt these practices, meal planning and grocery shopping will become valuable allies in your diabetes management journey, empowering you to enjoy delicious, satisfying, and blood sugar-friendly meals each day.

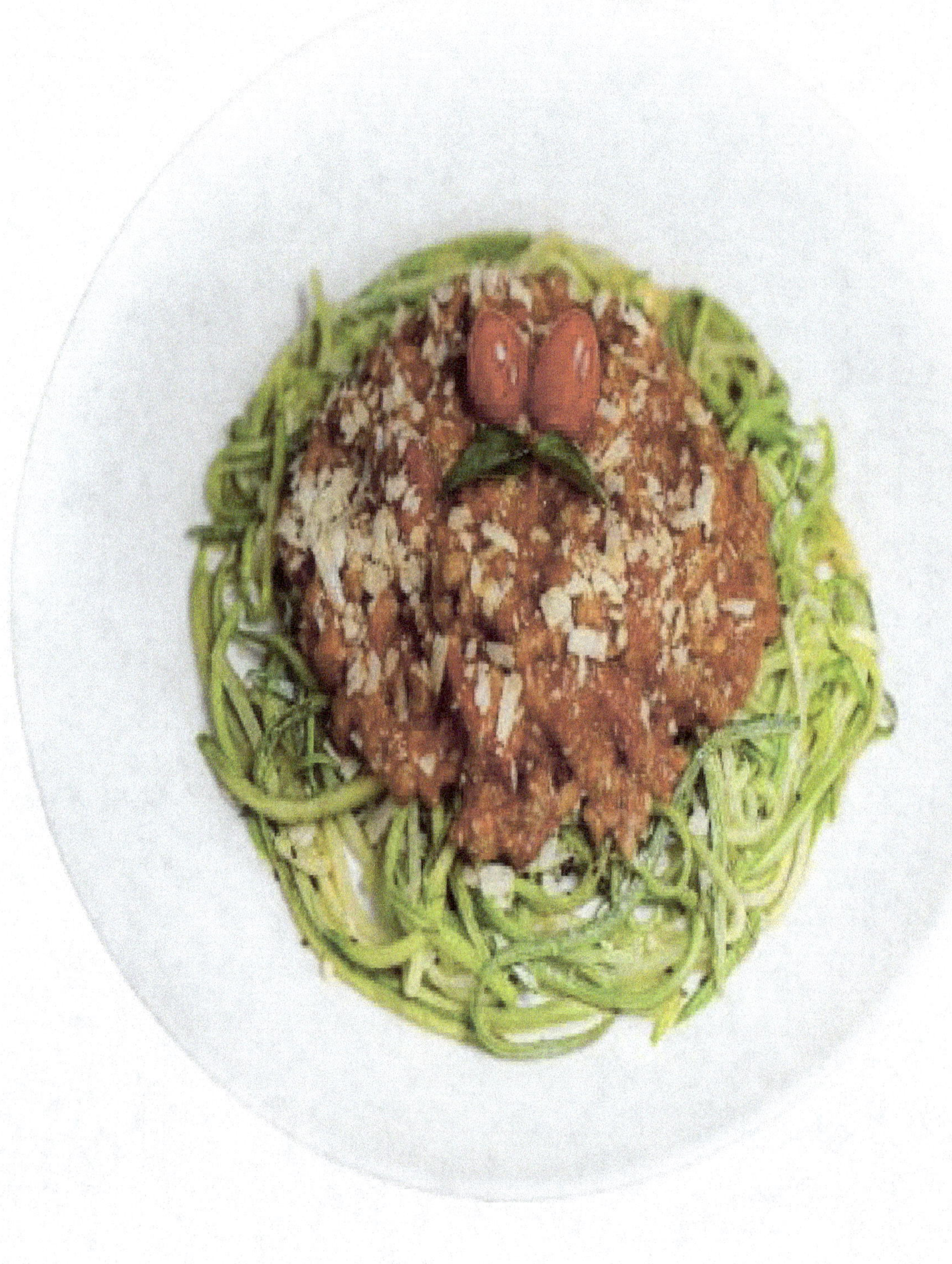